7 FOODS THAT LOWER BAD CHOLESTEROL (LDL) FAST AND NATURALLY

Fast and natural low density lipoprotein regulation

Julius Abdul

Disclaimer

It is not a complete guaranty that the recommendation in this book will lower your cholesterol, nor is it intended to replace your medical treatment.

You are aware that a consultation with a qualified healthcare professional, such as your doctor, is not intended to be substituted by reading this book. To be sure you are in good health and that following the information in this book won't hurt you, you should speak with your doctor or another qualified healthcare professional before starting any health modification program or altering your lifestyle in any manner, if after reading the information, you develop any strange symptoms.

Table of Content

Introduction

Ever get the impression that the cholesterol narrative is far more complicated than what we've been told? According to conventional thinking for many years, having high blood cholesterol levels is exceedingly harmful and can cause heart attacks, strokes, and even death. It must therefore be decreased by whatever means required. These methods include reducing your intake of cholesterol and saturated fat as well as using prescription medications that lower your cholesterol. Sounds familiar?

Well, some people stopped and asked a few straightforward questions: Isn't the human body much more complicated than this oversimplified answer suggests? Doesn't our health depend on multiple markers, such as total cholesterol? How and why did cholesterol come to be the bad guy? These are the important questions that I will address for you in this book.

It is true that cholesterol is generated as a result of some key factors and part of the factors that contribute to increase in cholesterol level in the blood vessel is your gene, this is what determine how your body processes the fat you eat and your family history. Familial hypercholesterolemia is a genetic condition that results in extremely high blood cholesterol levels and early heart disease. There is a 50% probability that you will also have familial hypercholesterolemia if one of your parents does.

Another aspect that needs careful attention is excess body weight, which raises the risk of high cholesterol.

Consuming alcohol excessively might raise cholesterol levels. Alcohol has calories in it that will cause you to gain weight.

The amount of cholesterol in the body is significantly influenced by age. The likelihood of having elevated cholesterol is higher in older adults. Women typically have lower cholesterol levels than men their age before menopause. This is so that women can metabolize the extra fat needed for pregnancy and delivery. However, the hormones stop secreting after menopause, which alters how a woman's body handles cholesterol.

Regular physical activity and exercise help your body burn fat and lower cholesterol levels. Sedentary behavior increases the likelihood of having elevated cholesterol.

Choosing the wrong foods can raise your cholesterol. The appropriate ones, though, might support bringing it back down to a healthy level. All the cholesterol your body requires is produced by your liver. However, some foods, particularly those heavy in saturated fat, might raise your blood cholesterol levels. The walls of your blood vessels can develop a waxy material from excess cholesterol. This hinders or lowers blood flow, which causes a wide range of issues.

Other illnesses like diabetes, liver disease, renal disease, polycystic ovarian syndrome, and circumstances that increase female hormones like pregnancy can also result in high cholesterol levels.

These are the principal contributors to cholesterol. You'll see that many of them are lifestyle variables if you pay great attention. You need to adopt more healthy behaviors and alter your lifestyle if you want to control your cholesterol. Let's discuss the seven foods that will reduce your LDL (bad) cholesterol.

What is cholesterol?

It is like a molecule that resembles wax and is produced in the liver, cholesterol can be found in the blood and all of the body's cells. Although it is not entirely bad, your body uses it to create hormones, vitamins, and new cells. Cholesterol can be divided into two fundamental categories, these are the High-Density Lipoprotein (HDL) and the Low-Density Lipoprotein (LDL).

High-Density Lipoprotein (HDL), also known as good cholesterol, takes in and transports cholesterol back to the liver, which ultimately excretes it from the body. HDL cholesterol reduces the risk of heart disease and stroke, but LDL, or bad cholesterol, has a high-calorie content that leads to obesity, diabetes, and heart disease.

There are also two different LDL varieties, but let's talk about cholesterol first. Since cholesterol cannot float down the bloodstream and is all fat soluble, it cannot mix with water. Therefore, when your blood profile reports your total cholesterol, you must understand that what they are measuring is all the cholesterol in the various protein shuttles, primarily HDL and LVL. There are other shuttles as well, but just keep in mind that these are the two main ones.

When you see a medical report of total cholesterol, what you're seeing is a combination of the cholesterol in the LDL and the HDL in general. Therefore, when we discuss HDL, which is known as the good cholesterol, we are referring to the HDL cholesterol that is moving from the arteries or cells back to the liver, and the LDL, which is regarded as the bad cholesterol moving from the liver to the cells or arteries.

What we'll be talking about in this section is crucial because, even though you might be worried if your LDL is extremely high, when you see the doctor to get your cholesterol checked, they almost always only test your LDL cholesterol and don't examine anything else that might be related to it. Since a very specific sort of LDL and a test that you would have to request are the true villains in the story of cholesterol and heart problems, it is crucial to realize that there are two different measurements for LDL.

This test, which stands for LDLP particle which is an Advanced Lipid Profile Test, will display the quantity and size of the particles. What is a particle, then? There are two particle sizes of LDL, the large buoyant version is called "pattern A," and buoyant means it floats to the surface. As was previously stated, it is a carrier that moves this cholesterol because it needs to have this protein little capsule to transport it. Therefore, it is these large fluffy particles that are floating through the bloodstream carrying cholesterol.

Then there are the little, dense particles that can get inside an artery since the inside of an artery is only around the thickness of a single cell. This is where the difficulty lies. The pathogenic LDL, not the huge buoyant LDL, but the small dense LDL, is where the issue originates. The key reason for concern should be the small dense LDL. The question I want to ask you at this point is, which LDL do you think has higher cholesterol? If you guessed large buoyant, you are right, so if your blood work results show that your LDL cholesterol is high, that information doesn't reveal what kind of particles you have more of.

It primarily provides information on the total amount of cholesterol, though some people with low levels of LDL cholesterol also have higher concentrations of the small, dense LVL particles, and many others with high levels of LDL cholesterol also have higher concentrations of the large, buoyant pattern type of LDL. Because it will offer you a complete view of what is happening, insist on receiving this Advanced Lipid Profile Test whenever you have your cholesterol examined.

Which Cholesterol-Rich Foods Should I Avoid?

Fast food

Regular consumption of fast food increases the chance of developing chronic diseases like obesity, diabetes, and heart disease.

Fast food also raises the risk of excessive levels of inflammation, abdominal fat, heart disease, and blood sugar regulation.

Processed meats

You should stay clear of processed meats like bacon, sausages, and hot dogs in your diet.
If processed meat consumption is not restricted, it can lead to colon cancer and heart problems.

Fried food

Fried meals are mostly linked to low-density lipoprotein (LDL), or poor cholesterol.

Trans fat

Trans fats and its high calorie content contribute to heart disease, diabetes, and obesity.
Vegetable oil solidifies at room temperature when hydrogen is added, which results in the formation of trans fats.
Food prepared with hydrogenated oil has a longer shelf life because this procedure is typically carried

out by businesses, which makes hydrogenated oil less expensive and less prone to spoil.

Because it won't need to be changed as frequently as other oils, the majority of restaurants utilize it in their deep fryers.

Small levels of trans fat are present in several dairy and meat products.

Trans fat can be found in a variety of food products:

- Commercially baked foods (cakes, pies, and cookies).
- Shortening
- Microwave popcorn
- Frozen pizza
- Refrigerated dough (biscuits and rolls)
- Fried foods (French fries, doughnuts, and fried chicken)
- Nondairy coffee creamer
- Stick margarine etc...

Small dense lipoprotein (LDL)

Now let's briefly go over more information regarding this tiny dense LDL, which is shown on your blood profile as "sdLDL." The first thing you should be aware of is that you will have higher levels of this profile—small dense LDL (sdLDL)—if you have metabolic syndrome, insulin resistance, obesity, or diabetes. You may also see this pattern—as was previously mentioned—if you have lower levels of LDLC cholesterol. Here, we are not evaluating the particles themselves but rather the cholesterol inside of these particles. This is crucial information for you to be aware of because there is sdLDL.

The tiny dense form of LDL that is involved in glycation is the atherogenic LDL. The term "glycation" basically refers to the process of mixing a protein with sugar, which renders the protein non-functional and causes issues with the proteins lining your arteries. Additionally, this type of measurement is connected to oxidation, which is another factor associated with inflammation and free radical damage. a favorable environment for the spread of bacteria, the formation of biofilms, tissue removal, and a cascade of other events, however, in addition to plaque buildup in your arteries, you frequently have biofilms, which are essentially microorganisms in calcium shells that tend to collect on the rough edges of your arteries brought on by oxidation or inflammation. As a result, small dense LDL is a strong 3x predictor of cardiovascular disease.

The other intriguing aspect of this is that while statin medications will lower your cholesterol, they do not affect this small dense LDL; in fact, they may even increase it. The main issue at hand is how to precisely lower the genuine bad LDL, which is the small dense version.

The best food to lower cholesterol

Well, there are some things you may consume that will benefit you. Each of the meals that will be mentioned has a considerable reducing effect on the tiny dense LDL, and they are all completely researched and proven foods.

Dr. Eric Berg DC, an internist with more than 20 years of experience in Solomons, Maryland, and an affiliate with CalvertHealth Medical Center, as well as the author of the best-selling book The Healthy Keto Plan and the Director of Dr. Berg Nutritionals, recommends the following foods in a YouTube video:

two avocados, because they are high in healthy fat, an extra virgin olive oil that you must make sure, is the real thing because there are many fake extra virgin olive oils out there. The following oil is fish oil, particularly cod liver oil, though you can also utilize fish oils. The omega-3 fatty acids, which include both EPA and DHA, come next; it appears that EPA is the one that has this reducing effect.

The next food is pistachios, which have also been shown to lower this small dense LDL. Next is dark chocolate, of which I would always recommend the sugar-free variety. Finally, there are almonds, which have also been shown to lower this tiny dense lipoprotein. Lastly, walnuts can aid in lowering harmful cholesterol.

Other natural ways to lower cholesterol

There are a few other pretty fascinating things that have to do with this subject as well. One of them is "Niacin," in particular the kind of niacin that induces blushing and has the power to transform from one particle size to another. These indicate that it can change your LDL cholesterol slightly lower while also switching from the small dense LDL to the large buoyant LDL, which is very good.

The next thing you could do is exercise, which will undoubtedly also help to lower this small dense LDL. If your problem is particularly stubborn, you could also try "Tudca," a very specific bile salt that helps the body get rid of extra cholesterol, Include extra exercise in your everyday routine by using the stairs instead of the elevator, parking farther from your workplace, going for a walk during breaks or downtime, and standing up more while doing chores like cooking or yard work.

You should also be aware that bile salts regulate cholesterol in the body bile salts are made from cholesterol, so if you are lacking in bile, such as if you have a fatty liver or no gallbladder, or if you have eaten foods that have slowed down the function of your bile ducts, that may be the cause of your high cholesterol. In this case, you should start taking bile salts, especially if you have a genetic condition that causes high cholesterol.

Please note, if you do have a genetic problem with your cholesterol and you want to do the ketogenic diet which I highly recommend with fasting, the thing you would want to do is not necessarily completely go low fat, you just want to avoid the extra fat that a lot of people take on the ketogenic diet which means you would not want to take the extra MCT oil and also don't want to start consuming the keto bomb treats filled with fat and butter, but you do want to increase the fish oils and the fish because that is not going to increase your problem. Additionally, sugar, especially fructose, is the worst food to consume because it tends to make problems worse.

This goes for all refined carbohydrates as well. Look for a means to quit smoking, these have immediate health benefits since it raises HDL (good) cholesterol levels. Your blood pressure and heart rate return to normal shortly after quitting cigarettes. Additionally, you will note that as your blood circulates, and your lung function improves over time, your risk of developing heart disease will vanish.

Although it is claimed that moderate alcohol consumption is associated with higher levels of HDL (good) cholesterol, this association does not support the recommendation of alcohol for non-drinkers.
Serious health issues like high blood pressure, heart failure, or a stroke can result from excessive alcohol consumption. Small weight loss adjustments add up to big results because being overweight raises cholesterol

levels. If you typically consume sugary beverages, try switching to water.

If you are curious to know how fasting can be your main strategy against cancerous cells, then search for "fasting; your main strategy against cancer, by Julius Abdul" on Amazon, and discover how fasting and another diet strategy can help prevent or cure cancer.

Conclusion

LDL is considered bad cholesterol, while HDL is considered good. However, there are two kinds of LDL. A specific type of LDL is the true villain when it comes to cholesterol and heart disease.

To measure this type of LDL, you must request a test known as an advanced lipid profile test. They are looking at the number and size of the particles that carry cholesterol with this test.

LDL is classified into two types or particle sizes which are; the massive buoyant (pattern A) and the tiny dense (pattern B).

Even though the large buoyant type carries more cholesterol, the small dense LDL particles are the ones to be concerned about because they can enter the arteries. Small dense LDL cholesterol is an excellent predictor of cardiovascular disease, because some people have low LDL cholesterol but a high number of small dense particles, this topic can be perplexing.

Others have high LDL and a lot of large buoyant particles. This is why it's critical to get an advanced lipid profile test to get a complete picture of what's going on.

Extra virgin olive oil, avocados, fish oils or cod liver oil, pistachios, dark chocolate (sugar-free), almonds, and walnuts are the top foods that lower bad cholesterol (small dense LDL).

Other natural ways to lower cholesterol include taking vitamin B3 (niacin), exercising, and taking TUDCA.